FOOD FIGHT!

Winning the Battle with
Food and Eating to
Achieve Sustainable
Weight Loss

BY LISA GOLDBERG MS, CNS, CDN

This book is dedicated to my loyal and hardworking clients who trusted me to help them with their lifestyle change and transformation. I am so proud of you. You really heard me and took to heart our conversations; you did the work, and came out happier, lighter and healthier on the other side. May you always hear my voice in your head.

"All the events you have experienced in your lifetime up to this moment have been created by your thoughts and beliefs you have held in the past. They were created by the thoughts and words you used yesterday, last week, last month, last year, 10, 20, 30, 40, or more years ago, depending on how old you are. "

~ LOUISE L. HAY

FOOD FIGHT

Lisa Goldberg MS, CNS, CDN - Nutritionist & Lifestyle Coach

Lisa Goldberg is a nutritionist and lifestyle coach with a Masters degree in Clinical Nutrition from New York University. She is a Certified Nutrition Specialist, a Certified Dietician/Nutritionist licensed by New York State, and Certified in Adult Weight Management by the ADA. Lisa served as the nutritionist on the New York Stock Exchange and created her own business HealthCoach that delivered healthy meals to traders from 2003-2013. She is also a personal trainer certified by ACE since 1994.

With more than 16 years of experience, Lisa specializes in weight-loss coaching around emotional eating, mindful eating, lifestyle and habit/behavior change - creating sustainable changes that enable her clients to lose unwanted weight for good.

> *"You can go on any diet under the sun. If you follow the diet plan you will lose the weight. But if you don't change the habits and behaviors that caused the weight gain to begin with, the weight will eventually come back".*
>
> - LISA GOLDBERG

Lisa believes that if you create an awareness about your habits and behaviors around food you can 'change your brain' and your relationship with food. You need to listen to the self-talk that happens internally and learn how to change it from a self- sabotaging voice into a voice that helps you reach your goals and maintain your ideal weight.

Many of Lisa's clients have described that before you change your internal voice, you need an external voice that keeps you accountable and honest about your feelings and ideas about food. A philosophy of everything in moderation allows Lisa's clients to reach their goals and not feel a sense of deprivation.

Lisa has her private practice on the Upper West Side in New York City and coaches clients virtually around the world.

She has created this book for people all over the world who want to gain knowledge about mindful eating and behavior change around food. It serves as a guide and a reminder of how to create sustainable weight loss.

Lisa Goldberg MS, CNS, CDN
www.lisagoldbergnutrition.com
212-920-0070
lisa@lisagoldbergnutrition.com

Foreword

These days, anyone looking for an authentic voice in the world of so-called diet experts is sure to be overwhelmed. One trip to the bookstore (virtual or brick and mortar) reveals volumes and volumes of how-to tomes – all of which promise to reveal the 'secrets' to losing excess weight and the 'tricks' to achieving your healthiest self.

As someone who has taken off over 250 pounds of excess weight (no, that number is not a typo – I once clocked in at over 450 pounds) and has kept it off for well over a decade, I can assure you there are no secrets or tricks. There are, however, plenty of carnival barkers who will proclaim they can sell you the 'formula' to fix whatever's holding you back from being your best – to which I advise: run (quickly in the opposite direction).

This is because the common sense and the tried-and-true weight loss advice most of us have heard throughout our lives is actually the smartest and most reliable path to wellness. The necessary feat, of course, is putting this common sense stuff to work in ways that complement our lives, rather than frustrate them (or lead us to stress-induced eating, which can pack even more pounds on top of the weight we initially wanted to get rid of).

It was, therefore, a very pleasant surprise to meet Lisa Goldberg for the first time – someone who embodied the picture of health, happiness, and fitness even before I knew what she did for a living.

And it was soon after meeting her that I realized Lisa does what she does as a calling.

Finding new strategies for enjoying healthier ways of living has always intrigued Lisa. And she gets excited when she gets the opportunity to share these findings with others. She truly cares about everyone looking to create positive change in his or her life. Lisa's compassion is palpable – and somewhat rare in the world of diet and health 'experts.' This is all because Lisa's more than authentic. She really gets it – and thus, can get to the heart of what might be holding someone back from reaching his or her full potential.

Still, Lisa's common sense approach is somewhat revolutionary – mainly because she delivers her easy-to-follow methods in an easy to embrace and compassionate way. Because she has worked with so many on their journeys to total health, she has a clear understanding of what's needed to win the battle of the bulge successfully.

It's through her wisdom that we can all develop new habits, re-train our daily behaviors and adopt the kind of mindsets that offer real freedom. And we can do all this without having to 'stop living life' during the transition (or, more accurately, during the transformation).

Lisa is all about living life to the fullest (no pun intended) and loving ourselves from the get-go. This means we can finally leave guilt and shame behind (the very things that have likely been holding us back all along). Her inspiring message and helpful strategies can offer all of us an escape from the on/off dieting cycle. She doesn't shroud her tactics and advice in hard to comprehend formulas or complicated recipes. She's about the real world living while using real foods as a tool. And yes, this even means there's room for our favorite treats along the way.

I'm thrilled that Lisa's Food Fight is delivering her message of hope, of wellness and of real results to people who may never be lucky enough to actually meet her in person or get to be coached by her. The information she provides in this book has the potential to bring self-empowerment to anyone who's truly ready to change his or her life for the better. This is why it's no secret (full circle!) that I'm one of her biggest fans – and always will be.

Gregg McBride
Screenwriter, Blogger, and Author
Weightless: My Life As A Fat Man And How I Escaped / Just Stop Eating So Much!

Preface

Calories in and calories out. Burn more calories than you consume. Protein grams, fat grams carb grams. Nutrition 101. I remember it well. When I first started my nutrition practice I followed this mantra. I gave my clients their nutrition plans (back then I referred to them as diet plans) and like any other plan, if you comply you will lose weight. Or so one would think. As I began to see more and more people come to my office, I realized that there was more to losing, or not losing weight than just following the plan that I gave them. It seemed the same conversations and questions kept coming up.

- I've gained and lost the same 20, 30 50 lbs, and I don't know why I can't keep it off?
- I don't know how it happened, but before I knew it, the weight came back.
- Why can't I stop eating at night?
- I have such cravings, I can't control them.
- I am good all day, and then I fall apart at night.
- I feel so stressed out I need chocolate.
- I eat, and I feel like I'm in a trance.

Does any of this sound familiar?

As I continued to work with people, it was clear that for many, the weight gain wasn't about the food. It was more about how they were conditioned growing up, their habits and behaviors around eating, the limiting beliefs they held about themselves and the stories they held onto in their heads based on these beliefs. They used food to stuff down and anesthetize their feelings; they used food as a reward for good and bad events or situations. They ate because they were lonely, sad, angry, stressed, anxious and any other feelings they didn't want to feel or deal with. There was no connection between hunger and satiety. I often heard "I don't know what hunger feels like."

I realized that to help people lose weight and keep it off I had to change more than just the food they were eating. I had to help them change their mindset and their relationship with food. Claiming to be a person that can help with weight loss, I knew that I had to have accountability and ethics around what I was selling. If I were to help people with nutrition without changing their mindset, there would be no integrity to what I was doing. I realized that I needed to create a program that was sustainable for people without the deprivation aspect.

So along with accountability and support, my approach for sustainable weight loss is first, eating healthy, unprocessed foods 90% of the time so there is no deprivation. Second, giving people the right tools and strategies to change their mindset and limiting beliefs that will lead them to change their habits and behaviors around food and eating. And last but not at all least, teach them how to incorporate better self-care into all aspects of their day-to-day life.

CHAPTER 1

My Story

My passion for nutrition didn't develop because I was overweight as a child or as a teen. Eating in my house was pretty standard. Sure we had Devil Dogs, Ring Dings and Hostess cupcakes in the house but food was not a 'thing' in my house growing up. We sat down as a family for dinner most nights during the week, except for weekends when my parents went out and usually left my sister and I with bagels and lox for dinner.

I'm sure my mother will deny it, but that's what I remember. Of course, there was the occasional fast food dinner during the week, McDonald's, Roy Rogers and Kentucky Fried Chicken, but most nights my Mom cooked dinner and I must say she was a pretty good cook. There was always a protein, some kind of vegetable and a starch of some description.

My sister and I were pretty good eaters. My Mom had a saying for new foods "try it, if you don't like it you don't have to eat it." I usually ended up liking it. It was a good start for a healthy relationship with food for my sister and me.

Typically after dinner, I went up to my room to do homework or in the den to watch TV with my Dad. Dessert was not an after dinner ritual in my house. When we were done with dinner, we were done. Occasionally there were snacks there if I wanted them but dessert did not "end the meal." Funny though, my Mom was a sweet eater but she was good with a piece or a bite and that was enough for her. In retrospect, that was very lucky for me. The behaviors and habits you learn around food and eating as a child often stay with you as an adult. It is imperative for parents to realize there is a family dynamic with food and eating and that children are a product of their environment.

My relationship with food, over-eating and nutrition began in college. I went to Syracuse University, home of buffalo chicken wings. I went to school in September a size 4/6 and weighed about 120 lbs. Two months later I arrived in Florida where my family spent every Thanksgiving. I stepped out of the airport where my parents were waiting and when my mother saw me said: "What the hell happened to you!" I was 15-20 pounds heavier and a size 9/10. I know to some of you reading this you may think 'What??? A size 9/10 isn't overweight.' But for a kid that was always thin and very athletic, it wasn't a body that I was accustomed to living in.

So how did I gain 15 lbs of pure body fat in two months??

Hanging out for hours in the dining hall eating (and overindulging) on brownies (a favorite of mine) and granola at various meals. Dominos pizza, chicken wings or subs ruled after partying at the bars at 2am and sometimes a combo of all. I guess I would be remiss if I didn't mention my drinks of choice that I discovered at school were pineapple bombers and mudslides. Calorically, both were a far cry from a light beer. Unfortunately as a new freshman, I didn't limit my nights out to the weekends.

It is not uncommon for teens or young adults, who go out on their own for the first time, to make bad choices about food. My diet was completely structured when I was living at home and now I had the freedom to eat and drink whatever I wanted and whenever I wanted. I had created a mindset for myself that, in retrospect, was highly detrimental to my health and well-being.

Getting back to Thanksgiving in Florida, I was miserable. I didn't want to go to the pool because I hated the way I looked in a bathing suit. None of my cute clothes fit anymore. Of course it had to be *that* year my parents decided to do something different and fly us to the Bahamas for a night. I didn't have any clothes that fit well or looked good. I actually fit into my Mom's clothes and she was a 10/12. I was beside myself. Even now I can remember the feeling. Ugh!

I began to diet while I was away. I ordered only seafood and used lemon on my fish and my salads. I didn't drink and upped the fruits and vegetables. I also bought a self-help tape. I don't remember exactly what it was called but I remember laying in the backyard listening to the tape in my Sony Walkman. (Yes, you read that right. A Walkman) Over and over I listened to 'you have a healthy, sexy body.' It worked for a while. By Christmas I had lost 12 lbs. I felt so much better.

Second semester freshman year I met a guy that I dated for the next three years. Though he was trim when we met, we had somehow plumped up together as the months went on. I guess it's more fun having someone to share your chicken wings with at 2am. You apparently feel less guilty when you have a partner in crime stuffing their face with you. I gained and lost the 12 lbs again by Spring Break and right after Spring Break gained it all back. I struggled with food, eating and weight like I had never struggled before.

One of my friend's during freshman year was majoring in nutrition. It was evident to me, as well as my other friends, that she had an eating disorder as she would only eat popcorn and apples and drink black coffee. She smelled the food she wanted to eat but wouldn't touch it. I, on the other hand, began this bad habit of overeating food that I liked and would find myself so full that I would make myself throw up. I remember once eating a whole box of Corn Bran cereal, I was so full I went to the bathroom and threw up. Unfortunately, that would happen now and again through my mid-20's. I never told that to anyone before as there is this feeling of shame that goes along with this negative behavior. I debated about putting it in this book, but since my clients are so honest with me, I felt that I should be just as honest. There is that integrity factor again!

So, by the time I got home for the summer, back up about 15 pounds, I was miserable all over again. I'd had it. I hated feeling fat. I hated being fat. I hated the way I felt in my body not to mention how I felt in my clothes.

As soon as I could I joined a Lucille Roberts (I'm really dating myself) and went on a strict diet. I had a job in Manhattan for the summer so when my Mom picked me up from the train I had her take me right to the gym. I also told her not to leave out dinner for me that I would prepare my own food (or not) when I arrived home. I watched everything I ate and read every health and fitness magazine that became my bibles for working out. I was diligent. I lost body fat and gained lean muscle. I totally redistributed my weight. I still weighed in the high 120's but I was a size 4.

My weight and my eating habits stayed pretty steady for the next three years while at SU. I left school in '86, started working at Bloomingdales in their retail training program, moved in with two roommates and once again had partners in crime and a bigger more exciting place to party-New York City. Needless to say, my weight fluctuated up and down. Every Sunday we pigged out on Chinese food and ice cream and every Monday we started a diet. I won't even begin talk about the amount of alcohol we consumed. My six pack abs that I worked so hard for were long gone.

Fast forward to 1993 where I was caught in the economic downturn and I lost my job (which was actually a blessing in disguise). As an unemployed person I spent a lot of time at the gym. One day I thought, 'I like this but what does one do to make a living in the fitness industry?' So long story short, in '94 I ended up at Equinox in membership sales and was then certified as a personal trainer. After training for several years I decided to go back to school to get my Masters degree in clinical nutrition and, as they say, 'the rest is history.'

I thought my story was important to this book because it explains how I have the empathy and understanding for my client's struggles with food, eating and weight gain. I laugh as I think how my clients always ask if 'I am in their head.' Although I didn't gain and lose weight my whole life, I did struggle with food and weight and experienced all of those terrible feelings you have about yourself. I get what it's like to pull every piece of clothing out of your closet and hate everything you put on. I feel your discomfort and your pain.

This is why when people come open to take the coaching and do the work, I can help them change their mind, their life and their relationship with food and eating.

CHAPTER 2:

Client Stories

Change & Transformation

I have worked with hundreds of clients in the 16 years I have been coaching clients on weight loss and nutrition. I usually get the call or email when a person is at the end of their rope. They just can't stand being overweight anymore and have come to realize that they need more than 'a diet.' The usual history is that they have gained and lost the same weight at least two or three times and have struggled with emotional eating and have spent most of their life of the proverbial diet roller-coaster.

It is funny how people will try roughly half a dozen or more quick fix diets, with the same results, before they realize that they need to create a sustainable change in their life for lasting weight loss. People will spend hundreds of dollars on shakes, fad diets, cleanses and drinks that they think will be the magic pill or potion that enables them to have the body they want without work. Yet, after years of empty promises, when they finally make lifestyle changes true results are attained. It begs the question, why do we easily spend money on gimmicks or the quick fix, but we question when we want to invest that money in ourselves for a lasting change? The work I do does not offer you a quick fix to weight loss. It offers you the promise that if you invest in yourself to learn how to change your mindset, break old habits and behaviors and change your relationship with food, you will have the tools to lose weight and sustain the weight loss.

Losing weight and, more importantly, sustaining the weight loss is about a lot more than just going on a diet. If it were that easy everyone would lose weight and not regain it. When you want to make permanent health, diet and lifestyle changes you need to be ready to do the mindset work that is required to help you make the mental shifts that will lead to a new way of thinking, which will then be followed by different actions. Just wanting to lose weight isn't enough. Change is a process that does not happen overnight. You have to be open to change and suggestions about how to make those changes. You have to be aware of the resistance that will come up in your brain that will try to keep you inside your comfort zone. You have to practice behavior change until it becomes just what you do without thinking so these new practices are woven into the fabric of your everyday life. It is about rewiring your brain.

I often use the analogy of learning to play the piano. You don't just decide one day to want to play the piano. You need to take lessons to learn the notes and chords, and then you have to practice. You have to repeatedly practice until you know the notes and chords by heart, and your brain and fingers know what to do without looking at the music any longer.

Once you have the tools to change how, when and why you eat, you need to continue using those tools to develop sustainable new habits and behaviors that you do without thinking.

Habit: *an acquired behavior pattern regularly followed until it has become almost involuntary.*

Here are some clients I have worked with whose stories you may connect with.

Barbara

Barbara came to me in September. She was 59 turning 60, and she wanted to lose 30-40 lbs by her birthday in July. She had been on and off diets and gained and lost the same 30-40 lbs a few times. But inevitably she gained it back because she did not change her habits around food and eating. She just became an expert dieter. Barbara's issue was binge eating. She ate for every mood. If she was in a bad mood she went to the deli for king size candy bars, cookies or cupcakes. But she also went to the deli was she was tired, stressed, pissed or even happy because she 'deserved a reward.' Does that sound familiar?

Barbara started to follow the plan I wrote for her and sent me her daily food records. As we began to work together I determined that Barbara had a sugar addiction, which didn't surprise me since she told me that she was a reformed alcoholic. She had an addictive gene to start with so she just replaced the alcohol with sugar. I came to learn that reformed alcoholics tend to crave sugar in lieu of the alcohol.

Barbara had to work extra hard since this was a big issue for her. We worked on mindful eating, increasing her awareness around her choices and getting in touch with her hunger. When she felt the urge to binge she was to ask herself Am I Hungry? And if the answer was no, we came up with a game plan as to what she could do with the feelings she was not used to feeling. What was great about Barbara was that she was open. She heard everything I said, AND she wrote things down that resonated with her. She would repeat what I said to her in her head and used that voice to make better choices. She had her setbacks but she moved ahead. She started to exercise and got a walking buddy and even walked with or without her. By her birthday she had lost 26.4 lbs. She was thrilled and she felt great!!

A couple of months after her birthday Barbara then decided that she could go it on her own. She took a four-month break in the fall and gained some of the weight back. She admitted she had stopped using her tools consistently. To maintain her weight loss, she needed to continue using the tools and strategies she had. We started to work together once again and refocused on getting her mindset back on track. She decided to hire someone to cook for her and her family once a week and prep meals for the remainder of the week. Barbara knew if she had what she needed it would be easier for her to stay the course. When I last checked in with her she was doing great.

For Barbara, more important than the weight loss were the changes she incorporated into her life and how much her mindset had changed. These changes would help her keep the weight off in the long-term.

Diane

Diane and I started working together in late December. I had rolled out a special promotion online that Diane had enrolled in. It was a 12-week program. Diane was a psychoanalyst in her mid- thirties. One of her goals was to lose 30 lbs. When she filled out her pre-consult questionnaire she told me that her biggest goal was to 'not have an emotional relationship with food and to be able to stop eating when she is no longer hungry.' She wrote "I have a tendency to eat more than I should when I am bored, lonely or sad. I'd like to tolerate the feelings that come up when I usually turn to food". This is from someone who helps others manage their emotions. It just goes to show that it doesn't matter what you do or who you are. When you have a deep- rooted relationship with food and eating, you give food the power to change how you feel.

Diane, like so many of my other clients, had been on and off Weight Watchers for the last five years before our meeting. My goal when I work with ex WW clients is to get them out of the dieter's mentality where there is a significant focus on counting points and calories. Who on earth wants to spend the rest of their life living this way? Although this type of program has it's benefits in the short term, it is not a sustainable way to live and will not help you maintain a healthy weight or relationship with food.

So the work began. I gave Diane her plan which, being a single thirty-something in New York City, included the leeway to go out for dinner a couple of nights a week and have some cocktails.

The work that I do is NOT about being on a diet. It is about finding a way to eat in the life that YOU lead. I used to be the nutritionist on the floor of the New York Stock Exchange and for ten years delivered healthy meals to traders outside the Exchange. There was NO WAY I could tell any of those guys I used to coach that they had to pass on their steak dinners and skip the martinis. I had to help them incorporate it into their life and still be able to lose weight.

Diane and I had ended up working together for a year not just 12 weeks. She was an excellent client. She took the coaching and each week applied the strategies that we talked about around her emotional eating into her life. Diane had many ah-ha moments especially around eating and dating. She would want to eat when she felt happy with her dates, and then she would want to eat when she was waiting for the text or phone call and her anxiety around 'what if he doesn't call' would start to set in.

Then there was what to do when she was on the date. To drink or not to drink? Diane could've very easily convinced herself that she needed to drink on her dates to have a good time or relax. But she changed her 'I CAN'T because' statement to an 'I CAN because' statement. I was so proud of her when she managed her mindset and realized it was OK if she decided not to. She knew her goal and her self-care was important. She made a choice based on what she thought and didn't worry about what someone else thought. I want to share with you Diane's testimonial.

I worked with Lisa for one year and as trite, as it sounds, the experience was life changing. In that year I completely changed my relationship with food – it is no longer a source of obsession, anxiety or stress for me. I have also lost 20 lbs and am happily and easily maintaining my goal weight. Lisa's approach is different from other diet plans. Rather than giving me a prescribed list of foods, making me count calories or depend on my willpower, Lisa taught me how to listen to my body and adopt healthier, more balanced habits and behaviors. With her guidance, I consistently lost weight without feeling hungry or deprived. I learned how not to eat emotionally and how not to use food as a source of entertainment. I'm off the roller coaster of thinking regarding 'good days' and 'bad days' with my eating habits. I eat without any residual guilt. I see the results of my year with her, not only in my weight but in my actions. These days, I can sit on the couch and watch TV without it occurring to me to make a trip to the fridge. I order whatever I'm craving at restaurants, but easily leave food on my plate. I can turn down delicious desserts because I'm full without getting cranky about it. I can get myself to the gym in the morning, even if I'm not in the mood. Food is no longer the focus of my thinking, and it's a relief. All that time I spent worrying or feeling guilty over my diet, is now spent in more productive ways. And I'm grateful.

It's important to mention that in addition to her extensive knowledge, Lisa is a pleasure to work with. She is non-judgmental, understanding, supportive and available. I couldn't have been happier in my experience with her. If you're unhappy with your relationship with food and are looking to make a real, sustainable lifestyle change, I would absolutely recommend her.

Diane lost 20 lbs during our work together. The last 10 lbs didn't really matter to her because she felt AWESOME in her body.

Like with all my clients when they reach their 'I feel good weight.' I give them a 4lb range to live in. For those who watch the scale, they know when they are getting to their high end of happy.

And you should know that I know what you were thinking a minute ago. 'Only 20 lbs in a year'!!!???

What you have to remember is Diane was learning how to change her habits and behaviors while she was losing the weight. She was learning and living how NOT to be on a diet.

* One side note about the scale. When I work with clients they have the option to weigh, not weight or step on backward so only I know the number. This is because so many people tie their self-esteem or failure and success to the number on the scale. I have a few clients that I've worked with for over a year. They have lost over 20 lbs and have no idea what they weigh. They only pay attention to how they feel in their body and their clothes.

I do not have a scale in my apartment. My jeans tell me everything I need to know.

Lara

Lara, a woman in her early 50's, came to me ready to do anything she needed to do to lose the weight for good. She was 30 lbs overweight and wasn't feeling good about the skin she was in. She was willing to invest in herself as she was tired of gaining and losing weight and wanted to stop yo-yo dieting. She was also peri-menopausal which presented an even bigger weight loss challenge as she was on hormone therapy. She told me she hadn't had an issue with weight until she hit her 30's and 40's.

Before she came to see me, she had tried Jenny Craig, Weight Watchers, South Beach and one or two other diets. Any weight that was lost on these plans came back as Lara just changed the food she was eating and nothing else. She went 'on' a diet and when she reached her goals she went 'off' her diet and the cycle continued.

Lara was at an advantage when we started to work together as she was doing regular exercise. She did stair climbing races around the city so to train for this she climbed stairs at least a couple of times a week. Lara's obstacles were similar to many of my other clients; mental or emotional stress, a sedentary job, lots of extra food at work and difficulty finding time to prepare healthy meals or snacks.

As we started our work together we focused on her changing how and what she ate and her habits and behaviors around food. Lara had friends in the city but often spent time after work by herself ordering in food and watching TV. Many a night after she was done eating, she would hear the leftover Chinese food calling her name. More often than not she couldn't quiet her mind from knowing the food was in the fridge until she just went back and ate it. That voice was in part loneliness and in part other emotions that she was trying not to acknowledge.

Once we started our work together Lara was great at sending me her food records. I encourage this as it helps me help my client stay on track in between our visits. Lara started to do the work by becoming mindful and paid attention to her choices. Week after week the weight started coming off. It's not to say that, at times, she didn't give in to emotional eating. Lara also realized that she often used food as a reward. She began to sign up for more climbing races. A couple of months into our work she competed in a race and did really well. After the race, she went out with friends and rewarded herself with a big meal. Needless to say, she didn't feel so well after as her body was used to eating cleaner, healthier food. As it turned out, she felt regret with her decision. Here she just accomplished a significant feat that she worked hard for and her reward was food. Unhealthy food. What kind of a reward was that??

It was a lesson learned for her. Lara continued to lose weight. As she lost weight she felt more confident in herself. She began to take spinning classes where she met friends and she also started to run some road races. She lost her 30 lbs in just over six months. And as a side note...the next time Lara did great on one of her competitive climbs she went out and bought herself a Tiffany wallet as a reward. Every time she reached for that wallet it reminded her of her accomplishment. Now that's a REAL reward!

CHAPTER 3:
Readiness for Change

"The key to change... is to let go of fear."
~ ROSANNE CASH

I can't tell you how often I get an email between 11 pm and 2 am from a potential client. It's usually at this time of night where people are alone with their thoughts; the most vulnerable, and often have just had some emotional or binge eating episode when they finally break down and reach out for help.

So often people are ashamed that they can't do it on their own. I had taken a survey of my community and asked the question 'what's stopping you from losing weight.' More than 50% responded- I know what to do I just can't do it.

I work with intelligent, educated women and men who have a handle on most aspects of their life except for food and eating. Some of them run multi-million dollar companies and yet how, what and why they eat is out of their control. They are the hardest on themselves since they are used to being successful in what they put their mind to. Changing your relationship with food and conquering emotional eating has nothing to do with how smart you are. One client once declared, "I have three degrees on my wall and yet I can't do this". It's because it's all deep-rooted in emotion, not logic, and based on old habits and behaviors around food and the limiting beliefs you have about yourself.

I have found that when people decide they are ready and wanting to lose weight they focus on just changing the food that they eat and exercise more. After all, for years we've heard it's about calories in vs. calories out. Eat less and exercise more. But, all calories aren't created equal so what you eat matters. You can't out-exercise a bad diet, and you cannot lose weight and keep it off if you do not also become mindful, change your habits, behaviors, your mindset and your relationship with food. This is the missing piece to the puzzle that doesn't get addressed as you go on diet after diet. Your food changes but these variables remain the same.

I have had clients come into my office thinking they are ready to change but in reality they were not. One client, I will call her Beth, came into my office wanting to lose some weight but mostly develop a routine way of eating healthy rather than waiting until she was starving and then make bad choices. She committed to working together for six months to help her create these changes. After one week she emailed me to say this wasn't the right thing for her because all she did was think about food and what she should be eating. I reassured her that this was part of the process until she developed new habits and her routine. She came back in for our next meeting, and we discussed what she was feeling. All seemed ok until the following week when, once again, I received an email saying that she just couldn't do it. As ready as she thought she was she gave in to the resistance that she was experiencing. Her brain was throwing up an S.O.S that this was going to be hard. Her fear got in the way, she reverted to the place of least resistance and she went back to the safety of her comfort zone.

Another client, I will call Betty, thought she was ready to create change. Betty wanted to lose 50 lbs. We spent six months together. Each week we discussed the obstacles that kept her stuck and made a plan for what she would work on. Each week Betty had a reason why she couldn't do it. She rarely sent me her food records because she was embarrassed she wasn't doing the work. She was ashamed that she was still overeating at night so she stayed in hiding. Not just from me but from herself. By not writing it down she didn't have to face it. This was her way of self-sabotaging.

Then there was Judy. Judy called because she felt that she was ready to get started but she just needed that extra push. She had a million excuses why she couldn't get started. She used being busy as one of her reasons. Her daughter was going off to school and she knew that it would be 'her' time soon to start paying attention to her needs so she could start to lose her last 15-20 lbs. One of her excuses was she needed to spend more time with her daughter before she left. Judy knew what she wanted to do, but she said "it was hard to put 'it' in motion. When I asked her what the 'it' was, she had no answer. The IT was HER. She couldn't put herself in motion to start to do for her own self as long as her daughter was still at home.

Making the commitment to lose weight is hard. Making the commitment to lose weight and focus on changing your habits and behaviors is even more challenging and takes a lot of mental and emotional work. You have to be ready to stay committed to your goals and yourself. Consistency is essential to create a real habit and behavior change. Change and transformation is a marathon and not a sprint. When you fall, and you will, you have to brush yourself off and keep going.

Are you ready to create real change? Are you ready to finally lose the weight for good?

Prochaska et, al developed the 5 Stages of Change

Prochaska's Stages of Change

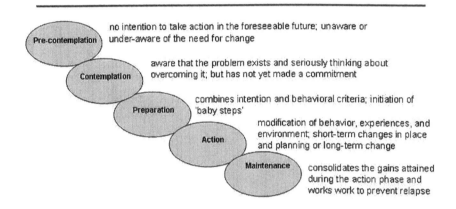

no intention to take action in the foreseeable future; unaware or under-aware of the need for change

Pre-contemplation

aware that the problem exists and seriously thinking about overcoming it; but has not yet made a commitment

Contemplation

combines intention and behavioral criteria; initiation of 'baby steps'

Preparation

modification of behavior, experiences, and environment; short-term changes in place and planning or long-term change

Action

consolidates the gains attained during the action phase and works work to prevent relapse

Maintenance

Data Source: Prochaska, J.O., Redding, C.A. & Evers, K.E. (1997). A Transtheoretical Model and Stages of Change. In K. Glanz, F.M. Lewis, B.K. Rimer (Eds.) Health Behavior and Health Education: Theory Research and Practice a (2nd edition) (pp. 60-84). San Francisco,: Jossey-Bass Publishers.

Slide Source: National Center for Cultural Competence, 2011

Stage One

Precontemplation - In this stage, people are not thinking seriously about any behavior change and are not ready or interested. In this stage, people tend to defend their current habits and behaviors and do not feel it is a problem. Some refer to this stage as being unready, resistant, unmotivated or being in denial.

Stage Two

Contemplation - In this stage, people spend some time thinking about their problem and can consider the possibility of changing but are still on the fence. People can spend a lifetime in contemplation. Though people are acutely aware of the pro's in creating positive change and they know they have a problem, they are not sure that the long-term benefits outweigh the short-term costs. In this stage, people are usually not planning to act within the next month. This step is also referred to as procrastination.

Stage Three

Preparation - In this stage, people have made a decision to do something. This is the stage where they know that the habit/behavior needs to change to order to find and alleviate the behavior/habit that causes or fuels their problem and pain. This is also an information gathering stage to find the best resource to help them make a significant lifestyle change. In this stage, people are ready to act within one month.

Stage Four

Action - This is the stage where people believe they have the ability to change and are taking the steps to get the help they need to change negative behaviors. They are open to seeking help. This is the stage where people make an overt effort to quit or change the behavior but are at the greatest risk for relapse. This is the stage where they make a commitment to themselves and develop a plan. This stage takes at least three to six months for change to take place.

Stage Five

Maintenance - The goal of maintenance is to maintain the behavioral/ habit changes that were made and to continuously practice the newly learned behaviors. It is important at this stage to remind yourself of the progress that you've done. People in this stage continually acquire new skills to deal with the new lifestyle change and avoid relapse. They can anticipate the situations in which a relapse may occur and prepare coping strategies in advance. They are aware that what they are striving for is worthwhile and meaningful. They are patient and recognize that it often takes a while to let go of old behavior patterns and continue to practice new ones. This stage extends from 6 months to an indeterminate amount of time after the action.

- What stage are you in?
- Are you ready to commit?
- Are you ready to change the way you think?
- Are you ready to change your relationship with food?
- Are you ready to do the work?

Being ready isn't about willpower. Willpower will only sustain you for so long as you probably have experienced in the past. Being ready is about focusing on your mindset. Change is a step-by-step process. It takes time. You can't expect to change your way of thinking and being around food and eating in a short period. This is why diets always fail. You either don't give yourself enough time to create real change or, when you do lose the weight, you go back to your old habits and behaviors. You have to allow yourself the time and be kind to yourself in the process. You have to be patient with yourself, and you have to be able to forgive yourself. How often have you started a new diet, eaten something you wished you didn't and then spent hours beating yourself up afterward? What if, rather than mentally beating yourself up, you forgave yourself and thought about what you could have done differently?

I often tell my clients, rather than sit in the remorse and regret, remember the feeling they had for making the choice that they made. If they felt bad about it, use that memory to contribute to making a different choice the next time. After all, why would you intentionally inflict pain on yourself now that you are acutely aware of the outcome? This will allow you to change the behavior if there is a next time.

CHAPTER 4:

Getting Started on Changing Your Habits and Behaviors

"You leave old habits behind by starting out with the thought. 'I release the need for this in my life.'"

~ DR. WAYNE W DYER

Being Planned and Prepared

The first step to change what, how and why you eat is to plan and prepare. Since the goal of all this change is sustainable weight loss, being planned and prepared for all of your meals and snacks is the most important step in the process. As you will see in Chapter 6, I included some quick and simple meal ideas, and in Chapter 7 some healthy recipes for breakfast, lunch and dinner. Whether you use my suggestions or you have your own plan that you like to follow, having what you need in the house and at work will help ensure that you make good choices. If you have what you need you can't/won't make a bad choice.

I had a client named Jill that I had been working with for months. She kept putting off getting to the grocery store because she was so 'busy.'

As it turned out, this was a recurring pattern for her. There was always something or someone more important that took priority over her own needs.

Part of making a lifestyle change is to learn how not to be too busy for you.

The truth is, we all find time to do what's important to us. When she finally got to the grocery store to have what she needed for breakfast, lunch, dinner and snacks, she came clean and admitted how much easier it was for her to make a healthy decision on what to eat since she had what she needed. It is work to make this a routine in your life, but it is work that you will benefit from for the rest of your life.

For this to become routine you have to take the action steps to create a new method of doing things. For Jill, it was finding the same one or two days during the week in which she would get to the store. Writing what you need to do on your calendar at a particular time will help to ensure that the task gets done. When you schedule a doctor's appointment you don't just decide you don't feel like going and not show up. Of course not! You schedule everything else that needs to get done around the doctor's appointment. You have to consider your needs to be just as important as getting to the doctor. That includes your exercise time, going to the grocery store, prepping food in advance and anything else that you need to do to take care of yourself and create your change.

My advice is to plan in advance. Whether it's a few days in advance or even the night before. Often (but not always) we know our schedules ahead of time. Take the time to look ahead to see what your week is like. Will it be routine, will you be out and about most days, do you have office meetings or are you traveling for business?

Do you need to bring lunch in case you are stuck in several meetings? If you are traveling, what snacks can you pack to be sure you don't get too hungry? It's difficult to stick to making healthy choices when you're starving. Real hunger doesn't feel good. Be sure to have what you need so your blood sugar doesn't drop leaving you hungry and cranky otherwise known as 'hangry'.

Awareness of habits, old patterns and triggers

The next step is to develop an awareness of what your habits and behaviors are around food and eating. Especially creating an awareness of that voice in your head. I always say there are two voices. The first is that old familiar voice that leads you down the rabbit hole. You know that voice. The one that is always saying 'I don't care, I want it' or 'I'll start again tomorrow.' Then there's the other voice, the logical voice in your head that will never steer you wrong if you listen. That's the voice that always gets pushed to the back because you are so used to listening to that old, more familiar voice.

Part of the awareness is becoming cognizant of what that voice is saying. What is the conversation in your head? Pay close attention to the messages you keep giving yourself. What I hear most from clients -

- I don't care
- What difference does it make
- It's going to make me feel better
- I'll worry about it tomorrow
- I'll show you
- Don't tell me what to do
- And the most popular one of all...Fuck it!

This usually gets an ah-ha response when I ask 'what is the **'it'**? Everyone sits there looking a little dumbfounded for a minute, and then I fill in the blank. There is no 'it.' The IT is YOU. Since I am pretty

27

direct in my coaching, I let them know that when they want to emotionally eat they may as well say 'fuck me, I don't care about me.' because there is no IT. This tends to make an impact.

These messages are the most common that I hear. All of your messages hold information about your patterns and beliefs around food and eating. Begin to ask yourself, 'Is this the truth?'

Once you start to pay attention to the messaging you give yourself, you then become aware of your habits and old patterns. It is eye-opening when you do the work and have an ah-ha moment.

One of my clients, I'll call Rachel, had struggled with weight most of her life. Rachel was in her 40's. One day while we were on our call she started to cry as she had finally realized why she always sought out cookies or candy at work. She worked in an office where there were cubicles and she had no privacy. Often the other women she worked with sat around chatting and joking around while she was trying to do her job. She resented it to some extent because she felt if she joined in that she may get in trouble. She focused so much on what was going on around her and it caused her real irritation and annoyance. She would think to herself 'if I just got a cookie then I could focus better on my work.' It gave her a reason to get away from her desk. She created a story in her head around why she should eat cookies. The story was 'poor me' I deserve a cookie (or most likely cookies) because I can't concentrate and it's not fair that they are sitting around talking while I am trying to do my job.

When Rachel became aware of the messaging in her head and why she kept trying to justify eating junk at work it was easier for her to change the behavior.

Here is what Rachel emailed me about her becoming aware of her habits and old patterns.

"Working with you has really made me think and peel back the layers and really get to know who I am and how I think.

I have printed out the meal plan that you posted- but I have come to realize I am a collector of information about some things... cookbooks, etc.

Most of the time I put the info (from you and in other things in my life) in a nice folder or notebook and think someday I'll do this or follow that... and I like reading posts on FB, but I have actually to do the things that are suggested.

I like the getting prepared part, but I need to do the follow through on things... and I what I am learning about myself is that if I think I won't do good or succeed at something or it might be difficult or unpleasant or a lot of work – I procrastinate or become lazy about it and not want to do it. I get caught up in the details being done correctly and need just to let it go (cooking my meals or whatever it might be) and so what if it is not perfect. At least I am doing it....

I really like your post today about the BS stories we tell ourselves that prevents us from our goal...that is me. Before working with you I wouldn't take ownership of that but you are getting through to me that I need to 'own it' and I have to do something about it and not be in victim mode or play the blame game."

Once you become aware of your habits and old patterns, it is easier to begin to start to change them.

Another part of becoming aware is noticing what your triggers are. Who, what, where and when are all factors to consider when trying to recognize your triggers.

Charles Duhigg, the author of *The Power of Habit,* created a flowchart on How to Change a Habit.

Let's say you want to stop eating at night after dinner. This particular habit is a prime cause of weight gain for so many.

First, there is the cue. When you feel the urge for your habit   ask yourself:

- What time is it?
- Where am I?
- Who else is around?
- What did I just do?
- What emotions am I feeling?

Second, there is the reward. What craving do you think your habit is satisfying? Is there a physical hunger?

Test the theory. Substitute another reward. For example, instead of reaching for the cookies make a cup of tea. Note if the craving is gone. If yes, then you were not really hungry, but the cue made you think of the cookies. If the craving is still there, try another substitute like going for a walk or taking a hot shower. If you are truly not physically hungry try another alternative until the urge passes.

The third step is the routine. Now that you've identified the cue and the reward you need to find a new routine. This new routine is what I call your Plan B. Each time you have an urge to eat after dinner when you are not hungry, repeat your Plan B until it becomes automatic when you feel the urge to eat.

Establishing self-talk

This is a big one. I am always asking what your self-talk was when a client tells me they were stress eating or mindless eating. I know there is always something going on up there as most, if not all, of the people I work with are chronic yo-yo dieters and emotional eaters.

Unless you are literally sleeping and eating there is some voice chattering away in your head. This is super important to pay attention to because this is the tape that typically plays time after time when you want to eat your feelings.

The first question you need to start with when you are not thinking about eating a meal or a snack is **AM I HUNGRY?** It is important to determine if you just feel like eating or you have real hunger. One of my tricks to identify hunger is to use a Listerine strip. If you think you feel like eating, or you are experiencing some emotion that makes you want to eat, pop a Listerine strip in your mouth. You will not want to put something else in your mouth since nothing really tastes good after one of those strips. Once the taste goes away if you are truly hungry you will still feel hungry. Using a strip or even brushing your teeth will give you time to pause and determine if you are really hungry. If you are then eat something small if it's not mealtime. Hunger doesn't feel good. So if it's late, eat just enough to get rid of the hunger.

Other questions and thoughts for your new self-talk-

- 'Is this the best choice I can make for myself?'
- 'Will this make me feel bad longer than it will make me feel good?'
- 'Will eating this change the situation?'
- 'It's just food. It doesn't have the power to change how I feel.'

This thought is important to sit with. Food doesn't have any power to change anything but your health and your weight, and it could be in a good way or a bad way. Logically, you know that when you emotionally eat you have conditioned yourself to believe that the food will give you comfort. Usually the thought is 'at least I have this.' But the truth is, emotional eating only fuels the bad feelings you already have. I describe it as adding coal to a furnace. As long as you continue to feed the flame, the flame remains. Only you have the power to make yourself feel better. You either implement your Plan B or sit with the discomfort and wait for the feeling to pass. Feelings are temporary and they will pass.

I can't emphasize enough how important your self-talk is. Establishing questions or mantras for yourself will make you better equipped to react in those moments you are triggered. When you are triggered, it's typically that old familiar voice that you immediately hear inside your head. When you hear that old voice playing that same old tape be prepared with the question 'is that the truth?'

- 'I want it now; I don't care.' Is that the truth?
- 'Well, at least I have this.' Is that the truth?
- 'I'll never lose weight anyway.' Is that the truth?

Do you see where I am going with this? You have to change that old tape in your head. It will bring you down the rabbit hole every time. This is what I mean when I say you have to rewire your brain. You have to reprogram your way of thinking and get rid of your old story and limiting beliefs about yourself.

Another question for your self-talk is 'what is the benefit if I eat_____ and what is the benefit if I don't'? You fill in the blank.

Mindful Eating and Eating with Awareness

I believe weight loss and long-term maintenance is not possible without becoming mindful about what, when, where and why you eat. I believe one of the main reasons people tend to regain the weight that they've lost after going on a diet is that they stop being mindful. Once the weight loss goal is achieved you can't just stop doing what helped you to lose the weight. Hence, being 'on' and 'off' a diet. Once you hit your goal weight, or even just start feeling better in your body, it is even more important for you to stay mindful of your food choices, portions, emotional eating and your hunger and satiety to be able to sustain the weight that is lost.

Here are The Principles of Mindful Eating as created by The Center for Mindful Eating. www.thecenterformindfuleating.org.

Becoming familiar with the principles of mindful eating can deepen your understanding of this concept.

The Principles of Mindfulness:

- Mindfulness is deliberately paying attention, non-judgmentally.
- Mindfulness encompasses both internal processes and external environment
- Mindfulness is being aware of what is present for you mentally, emotionally and physically in each moment.
- With practice, mindfulness cultivates the possibility of freeing yourself of reactive, habitual patterns of thinking, feeling and acting.
- Mindfulness promotes balance, choice, wisdom and acceptance of what is.

Mindful Eating is:

- Allowing yourself to become aware of the positive and nurturing opportunities that are available through food selection and preparation by respecting your own inner wisdom.
- Using all your senses in choosing to eat food that is both satisfying to you and nourishing to your body.
- Acknowledging responses to food (likes, dislikes, or neutral) without judgment.

- Becoming aware of physical hunger and satiety cues to guide your decisions to begin and end eating.

Someone Who Eats Mindfully:

- Acknowledges that there is no right or wrong way to eat but varying degrees of awareness surrounding the experience of food.
- Accepts that their eating experiences are unique.
- A mindful eater is an individual who, by choice, directs their attention to eating on a moment-by-moment basis.
- Gains awareness of how they can make choices that support health and well-being.

Mindfulness helps you to be present at your meals. Focusing on how the food tastes and smells. Good tasting food does bring pleasure. So when you are eating, focus on getting the pleasure you are seeking from your food. My clients hear me say ALL of the time; there is nothing you can't eat, and I mean that. From my point of view nothing is off limits, just how much and how often in seven days. This prevents feelings of deprivation. After all, I would never want to go through the rest of my life never having a brownie or a cheeseburger and fries and I would never expect my clients to either.

If you are going to eat a brownie or a hot fudge sundae, or whatever it is that is considered a splurge, get the pleasure from it that you are seeking. Savor it. If it is a mindful decision and not an emotional decision there is no guilt. Once you learn to be mindful around food and eating it will be easier to make a good choice. Everything you put in your mouth is a choice. No one is pushing the food down your throat.

Which brings me to one other thing to be mindful of. Those people who, knowingly and unknowingly, sabotage you. You know, those people that push food on you when you tell them you are watching what you're eating. There are those people that will want you to eat with them to alleviate any guilt they may feel if they indulge alone. And then there are those that don't have a weight issue and can't understand what the big deal is if you eat something you prefer not to eat. Don't eat to make someone else happy or because you feel uncomfortable saying 'no thank you'. The irony is so often people will eat something someone else wants them to try or share, then they feel good and you feel bad.

Practice Practice Practice

There's a reason why losing weight and keeping it off is so difficult. There is more to sustainable weight loss than just going on a diet. Changing what you eat is the easy part. Changing your mind and your habits and behaviors is the hard part. You have to learn how to operate entirely differently around food and eating. You have to change the way you think as your behaviors follow your thoughts. Long-term weight loss is achievable if you implement what you have learned so far and you continuously practice your new way of thinking and your new behaviors, until your actions become new habits that replace your old ones. So often people who go on a diet will work hard on diet and exercise, and as soon as they hit their goal weight or get close to it, they get what I call Cocky Dieters Syndrome. All of a sudden they think they are Teflon to calories and slowly begin to go back to their old way of eating. The mindfulness and mental and physical work that was exerted for the weeks or months they worked so hard to lose the weight, somehow no longer exists because the thought is it's no longer necessary. The task at hand has been accomplished. So as the weeks and months go by, little by little the weight creeps back on until one morning you get up freaking out and saying 'I don't understand how this happened. How did I gain this weight back'??

You stopped the routine you had established. You reverted to the place of least resistance when you were in a bad mood or perhaps even a good mood.

You never established a regular mindfulness practice, or if you did you didn't continue. You stopped paying attention to your hunger and satiety and you never changed your thoughts or your relationship with food. Only the food changed but your emotional attachment to it didn't.

If you want to lose weight and keep it off you need to establish a lifestyle and mindset around food and eating that works for you. Don't eliminate food groups from your diet if, in reality, you don't want to live without those foods. You have to create changes you can live with for the rest of your life or the weight will just come back.

You have to remember there is no perfect. There will be peaks and valleys, but as long as you keep rising and moving forward you will be able to sustain being mindful.

In March of 2016, I interviewed Dr. Elisha Goldstein on one of my tele-summits titled 'A Well Fed Mind.' Dr. Goldstein runs The Center for Mindful Living in West Los Angeles, California. During our interview he drew a diagram as we were addressing the practice of mindfulness. It was a simple drawing but it made a huge impact. I recall drawing it for one of my clients at the office one day and I could see the light bulb go off for her. This simple drawing showed her that there would be peaks and valleys in creating change and becoming mindful. But as long as she kept climbing back up and kept moving forward she was headed in the right direction.

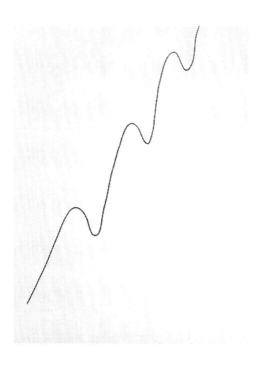

Practice your new way of thinking, practice your new behaviors, practice the new routine you created for yourself, practice your Plan B, practice being mindful and before you know it, you will have created new habits and a healthier emotional and physical lifestyle you can sustain.

"One of the massive imbalances in life is the disparity between your daily existence, with its routines and habits, and the dream you have within yourself of some extraordinarily satisfying way of living"

~ DR. WAYNE W DYER

CHAPTER 5:
Putting the Brakes on Emotional Eating

"If Hunger is not the problem, Food is not the Answer"
~ LISA GOLDBERG MS, CNS, CDN

When I start working with clients one of the first questions I ask is 'what do you want and WHY do you want it'?

The answer has to be bigger than I just want to lose X numbers of pounds and feel better. I ask them to go deeper. How would your life change if you created this transformation? What is your vision for your life? How would YOU change if you transformed and began to live your vision?

I ask them to do this because when it comes to emotional eating, when that feeling hits of wanting to eat to soothe those feelings they are trying so desperately to avoid I want them to recall their WHY.

Your WHY has to be so important that you realize that it is more important to you than that cookie, brownie or French bread. I want you to understand that you are trading in your WHY and your vision for your life for unhealthy food that WILL NOT make you feel better.

It will only take you further away from your goals, your dreams, and your WHY.

I want you to remember that *its just food*. Food has no power. It only has the power that you give it.

When you learn how to break the emotional eating loop you can take back your power from food.

Understanding the Loop

I am a big believer that when you understand what makes you operate the way you do, it is easier to create the changes you want to make. The more aware you are of your behaviors and understand those behaviors, the easier it will be for you to modify your behavior because you recognize it when it is happening.

When you understand the emotional eating loop the feelings you experience have less power over you. It's helpful to give names to each phase so they're easier to identify when they come up in your daily life.

Phases of the emotional eating loop

There are three main phases of the emotional eating loop: Trigger, Numbing-out, and the Aftermath

Trigger: A trigger by definition is -

> *"Anything, as an act or event, that serves as a stimulus and initiates or precipitates a reaction or series of reactions."*

A person, place, event, or even the time of day can cause a trigger. The trigger evokes an emotional response that can then create a physical response in the body. Your breathing may speed up or become shallow; you may start sweating. Emotionally, you might feel angry, sad or annoyed. The trigger is what sets your brain in motion to think about food and causes you to emotionally eat.

Numbing Out - There are many ways to numb out feelings we don't want to feel, but one of the most common ways is to eat foods high in sugar, carbohydrates and fat such as ice cream, cakes, cookies, chips, nuts, bread and so on. These foods are typically the food of choice that are used to numb out or anesthetize the feelings you don't want to feel. While you are eating these comfort foods you are just focused on the act of eating; you are not thinking about the feelings or the trigger that evoked the feeling. You are 'numbing' those feelings out, at least for the moment. This phase is usually followed by regret, remorse or shame leading you to the next phase.

The aftermath - The aftermath includes both emotional pain and physical pain. The regret, remorse and shame are just some of the emotional side effects of emotional eating. Negative self-talk also rears its head in this stage. 'I'm an idiot, I suck, I'm such a loser' are just some examples of critical self-talk I have heard over the years. The physical effects are the feeling of being over-stuffed, bloated and uncomfortable in your body.

4 Steps to Breaking the Loop

1. **Create Awareness -** Once you are aware of your habits and behaviors around food and eating the habits and behaviors will be easier to change. You also need to create an awareness of how your body feels. When we are stressed or anxious our body begins to get tense. Often, anxiety starts in the pit of the stomach and works its way up. Be aware of the stories that you tell yourself in these moments that can either bring you down the rabbit hole or lead you away from it.

2. **Address the trigger -** The best way to avoid the emotional eating loop is to address the trigger. What happened in the moment or

during the day. Who was/is there? Where are you? Addressing the issue often eliminates the desire to eat emotionally because you are acknowledging the feeling or feelings head on rather than trying to numb them out. Feel your feelings. You have to get comfortable being uncomfortable while you are acknowledging the feelings you 'want to eat.'

3. **Create a 'Plan B' of healthy habits and Self-Care -** Make a list of alternative things that you can do to make yourself feel better that doesn't involve food. I often recommend a cup of hot tea. You usually use both hands to hold the hot mug and you feel the hot liquid going down which is soothing. Take a hot shower or a bubble bath. Catch up on your favorite magazines, do a crossword puzzle, call an old friend, take a walk, do some yoga poses. Whatever it may be for you, make it part of your Go-To rather than head for the kitchen. The more you practice utilizing your Plan B, the more automatic it willbecome.

4. **Identify the root cause -** When we repeat our patterns that cause us pain it keeps us from getting where we are now to where we want to be. Getting to the root means asking ourselves some deep questions about why we do the things we do. That may mean going back to your childhood or part of your past that made you sad or perhaps you prefer to forget altogether. Again, when you understand the 'why' of your thoughts and behavior patterns they will be easier to change.

I fully acknowledge that this work is hard. But this work is the missing piece to the puzzle. If the answer to sustainable weight loss was to go on another diet, we would not have a society of yo-yo dieters or an obesity problem.

The work that I do can help you create real, consistent and sustainable change. I hope I have given you some of the tools and strategies that you need to get started on your journey to transformation.

CHAPTER 6:

Quick and Easy Ideas for Eating Healthy

"The first wealth is health"
~ RALPH WALDO EMERSON

I cannot write a book about sustainable weight loss without talking about food and what to eat. My philosophy on food and eating is that there is nothing you can't eat. That being said, I do believe in eating healthy unprocessed foods as the mainstay of your diet. I actually hate the word diet, but there doesn't seem to be another word when talking about how you feed yourself. I don't cut out food groups when I work with clients unless, along the way, I feel that something is preventing them from losing the weight, or there are foods that they cannot or prefer not to eat. I believe that if you eat well most of the time, you can eat crappy some of the time and it won't affect your weight. Remember when I spoke about eating well 90% of the time? That leaves you 10% to live your life without feeling like you can never eat anything unhealthy or fattening.

When I work with clients we focus on how much and how often in the course of seven days. This way there is room for indulgences one or two days during your week. This helps to prevent feelings of deprivation. I want to teach people how to eat in a way that is sustainable, and I find this philosophy allows you to eat without feeling like you have to be perfect. There is no perfect. There will be days, even after changing how you eat, that you will eat something and think 'Hmmm, I probably didn't need to eat that.' That's ok. Don't beat yourself up. Move on. You will have the rest of the day or the next day to get back to your new, usual way of eating.

Here are some ideas for breakfast, lunch, and dinner.

QUICK AND EASY BREAKFAST IDEAS

- 2 Hardboiled eggs with 2 Ryvita crackers and 1 orange.
- Fresh blueberries or 1 small banana with Natural Peanut butter on sprouted grain bread
- Plain Greek Yogurt crushed walnuts or almonds berries
- Natural Peanut butter or Almond Butter on sprouted grain bread and sliced apple.
- Cottage Cheese on sprouted grain bread or 100% whole wheat English muffin with sliced tomato. 1 piece of fruit.
- Omelet, add any vegetables with 100% whole wheat or Rye toast (or other high fiber bread). You can add some cheese if you desire.
- 100% whole wheat English muffin with ¼ sliced or mashed avocado with one sunny side or sliced hardboiled egg.

QUICK AND EASY LUNCH IDEAS

- Grilled chicken breast rolled in a whole wheat or corn tortilla with romaine, tomato, crumbled feta cheese, drizzle olive oil and vinegar. 1 Apple

- Tuna fish with a little mayo and mustard on sprouted grain bread w/ romaine and tomato. 1 cup cut cantaloupe.

- A Large mixed green salad with a variety of colorful vegetables. Add any protein like chicken, shrimp or hardboiled egg or egg whites. 2 T olive oil and vinegar or 2 T of any regular dressing. 1 cup berries.

- Fresh Turkey Sandwich on Ezekiel 100 % whole wheat or rye bread with avocado, romaine, tomato, hummus. 1 pear or small green salad. If you prefer not to use bread for your sandwich lettuce leaves make a great roll-up.

- 1.5 cups cooked brown rice pasta or whole-wheat pasta tossed with chicken (or any protein), cherry tomatoes, broccoli. Tossed with 1-2 T oil and balsamic. You can season with garlic powder and red pepper flakes depending on taste.

- Any non-cream based soup with one half of a turkey sandwich or a medium mixed salad with a variety colorful vegetables and 2 T any dressing of your choice.

QUICK AND EASY DINNER IDEAS

- **Stir Fry** –chicken, broccoli, red and yellow peppers, toss with 1 T sesame oil, low sodium soy sauce. You can add sesame seeds and red peppers flakes. Serve over brown rice

- **Turkey Chili**- ground turkey or chicken, canned plum tomatoes, chili seasoning, black beans, brown rice, add a mixed green salad w/ 2 T balsamic and oil.

- **Grilled Tuna or Wild Salmon**- Season either fish with a little salt and pepper and grill. You can also brush the fish with some pesto or drizzle on after the fish is cooked. Sautéed spinach and kale in chicken broth, shallots, garlic 1-2 T olive oil. Serve with quinoa on the side.
- **1.5 cups cooked whole wheat pasta** or brown rice pasta chicken, or 1 chicken or turkey sausage sliced, broccoli or spinach. Sauté vegetables in low sodium chicken stock and garlic. Small side salad w/ 2 T balsamic and olive oil.
- **Whole wheat tortilla Pizza** with shredded mozzarella cheese, zesty tomato sauce, with sliced mushrooms and/or spinach with a green salad on the side.

CHAPTER 7:

Healthy Recipes

"A healthy outside starts from the inside"

~ ROBERT URICH

These healthy and tasty recipes can also be found in my Free **Create Your Change Weight Loss and Motivational Guide** which you can download from my website www.lisagoldbergnutrition.com

---

BREAKFAST

Oatmeal Breakfast Bowl

Serves: 2

Ingredients:

- 1 cup steel-cut oats cooked according to package directions. *(Tip: You can cook ahead of time and double up the batch for a quick breakfast bowl during the week.)*
- A nice sprinkle of nuts and seeds (pumpkin, sunflower, almonds, chia, walnuts),any nuts/seeds you like or have on hand)
- ½ cup berries
- ¼ cup for each bowl unsweetened almond milk (optional)
- Stevia or a little honey, to taste
- Dash of cinnamon (optional)

Directions:

- Combine all ingredients in a bowl and serve warm.
- Top with berries, a sprinkle of Stevia/honey and a dash of cinnamon.

Mushroom & Asparagus Frittata

Serves: 2

Ingredients:

- 1 cup sliced fresh mushrooms
- 1 cup asparagus spears, sliced diagonally into 2-inch pieces
- 1 green onion, white and green parts chopped fine
- Olive oil spray or 1 T olive oil
- Sea salt & fresh ground pepper to taste
- 6 egg whites lightly beaten in bowl
- 2-3 T chopped fresh basil (use 1-2 T dried if you don't have fresh)
- Fresh melon slices (Optional, for side garnish.)

Directions:

- Preheat oven to 350 degrees
- In a non-stick oven-proof skillet, heat oil and sauté mushrooms and asparagus until asparagus starts getting crisp (about 3-4 minutes.)
- Add in green onion and continue to sauté another minute.
- Salt and pepper then pour in the egg whites.
- Sprinkle the basil on top.
- Place the skillet into oven and bake for 5 minutes until center of frittata is 'set' and the edges pull away from the skillet.
- Remove skillet and slide frittata onto plate or cutting board.
- Allow to cool a minute then slice into wedges.
- Serve with sliced fruit, like melon

Organic Egg-Veggie Scramble

Serves: 1

Ingredients:

- 2 organic, cage free eggs or egg whites
- 1 T olive oil
- 2 T onion, chopped
- ¼ cup mushrooms, sliced
- ¼ to ½ cup spinach
- Fresh or dried chives (chopped, if fresh)
- Sea salt & pepper to taste

Directions:

- In a bowl, whisk eggs vigorously for 15 seconds
- Heat oil over medium heat.
- Add onions, cook for several minutes, making sure not to burn.
- Add mushrooms and spinach and cook for another minute.
- Stir in eggs and continue to stir in pan, scrambling all ingredients together until desired doneness.
- Add a little more olive oil during cooking if needed.
- Salt & pepper to taste and sprinkle on chives.

Note: Get creative and use fresh veggie ingredients on hand.

Easy Tofu/Seitan Scramble

Serves: 2

Make this your own by adding any veggies you like. This is a basic go-to recipe.

Ingredients:

- 1 block tofu, drained and pressed OR ¾ cup seitan strips, chopped into bite-size pieces
- ½ small onion, diced
- 1 clove minced garlic or 1 t garlic powder
- ½ green, red or yellow bell pepper, diced
- 2 T olive oil
- 1 T soy sauce (optional)
- 2 T nutritional yeast (optional)
- ½ t turmeric (optional)
- Salt and pepper to taste
- 2 whole wheat, whole grain or gluten-free tortillas
- 2 T fresh salsa (optional. for topping tortilla)
- 2 T shredded dairy or vegan cheese (optional, for topping tortilla)

If using tofu: Slice the tofu into one-inch cubes. Using either your hands or a fork, crumble it slightly.

Directions:

- Heat oil and sauté onion, pepper and crumbled tofu or seitan for 3-5 minutes, stirring often.
- Add remaining ingredients, reduce heat to medium and allow to cook 4-7 more minutes, stirring frequently and add more oil if needed.
- Season with salt and pepper to taste.
- Divide the mixture and wrap in a warmed whole-wheat tortilla.
- Top with salsa and cheese if adding.

Quick and Easy Huevos Rancheros

Serves: 2

Ingredients:

- 2-4 organic eggs or egg whites
- Olive oil spray (or 1 T olive oil)
- ½ cup whole grain or rice tortilla chips
- ¼ cup shredded Mexican cheese or vegan cheese
- 2 T sour cream (Optional)
- 2 T fresh, natural salsa (no sugar added)
- Hot sauce (optional)
- Chopped cilantro (optional)

Directions:

- Spray skillet with olive oil spray or coat with olive oil.
- Cook eggs to desired doneness (over-easy, sunny-side up, etc.)
- Sprinkle cheese evenly on both eggs and add pan cover to let cheese melt for a minute or so.
- Meanwhile, separate the chips onto 2 plates.
- Divide eggs on top of chips.
- Top with salsa and sour cream.
- Sprinkle a little hot sauce and/or cilantro if desired.

LUNCH AND DINNER OPTIONS

Super Salad

Makes 2 servings

Salads, and what you dress them with, are full of wonderful, nutritional ingredients that are vital to a healthy body. This recipe is a *guide*, but think about using up the odds and ends in the fridge. If you don't have exactly what's on the list, improvise! You could add some tuna, grilled chicken or beans for a protein punch.

Ingredients:

- 4-6 cups fresh salad greens like butter lettuce, red-leaf lettuce, spinach or romaine, mix it up!
- 1 small-medium handful of arugula or kale
- ½ avocado, peeled and diced
- ½-1 tomato, or hand full chopped cherry tomatoes
- ¼-½ medium cucumber, chopped into bite-size pieces
- 4 dandelion greens (optional)
- handful of shredded red/green cabbage
- ½ carrot, shaved with a vegetable peeler
- 3-4 chopped fresh basil sprigs
- 4-5 chopped fresh cilantro sprigs
- 1 t hemp seeds (optional)
- 1-2 T toasted sunflower seeds or almonds (spread on a baking sheet and roast at 300 for just a few minutes, they toast fast so keep an eye on them!) OR add them in raw.

Directions:

Get a big salad bowl with lots of room. Add the lettuce, arugula, kale, avocado, tomato, and cucumber and whatever other veggies you're playing with. Top with the dandelion greens, carrot shavings, and herbs. Sprinkle with the seeds and nuts. Lightly salt & pepper   if you like.

Drizzle the dressing (ideas below) directly onto the salad and toss. And voila! Your super salad is ready for you.

Dressing Ideas:

Apple Cider Vinaigrette:

- 2 T olive oil
- 1 T apple cider vinegar
- 1 T dijon mustard
- Whisk all together in a bowl until creamy.

OR:

Oil/Citrus Dressing

- 2 ½ T infused olive oil (basil, truffle, etc.) OR extra-virgin olive oil
- 1 ½ T balsamic vinegar
- Juice of ½ lemon
- Juice of ½ orange (or a little more lemon if you don't have orange)
- ½ t grated vegan Parmesan cheese (optional)
- Whisk together until creamy.

OR:

Avocado dressing

- 1 large ripe avocado
- 1 garlic clove
- ¼ t hot pepper flakes
- 2 T lime juice
- 2 t olive oil
- ½ cup water

Place all the ingredients in a blender and process until smooth. Adjust the amount of liquid to obtain nice creamy dressing. Enjoy!

Veggie Bowl With or Without Chicken

Serves 2-4 (depending on if being served as a main or side dish)

Ingredients:

- 1 cup quinoa or brown rice, cooked according to package directions *(Tip: cook in vegetable broth instead of water for fuller flavor.)*
- 1-½ cups broccoli florets, chopped
- 1-½ cups cauliflower, chopped
- 1 cup carrots, peeled and diced
- 1 cup spinach, coarsely chopped
- 1 red pepper, chopped (you can use yellow or orange peppers as well, or a mixture)
- ¼-½ cup fresh parsley, finely chopped (optional but so healthy)
- ¼ to ½ cup sunflower seeds, pumpkin seeds or a mixture
- Juice of ½ lemon
- Sea salt and pepper to taste
- Drizzle of olive oil
- Dash cayenne (optional-if you like a little kick!)
- ½ to 1 lb cooked, diced organic chicken breast (Optional, if you want the extra protein or making as a heartier meal.)

Directions:

- Steam broccoli, carrots, and cauliflower for 5-7 minutes, (depending on your desired tenderness) adding in peppers for the last 2-3 minutes.
- Chop the spinach and parsley.
- In a large mixing bowl, toss together cooked quinoa or brown rice, steamed vegetables, spinach, red pepper, and parsley.
- Add the raw seeds and drizzle with lemon juice, oil and salt & pepper to taste.
- Serve cold or warm

Curried Tuna or *Mock Tuna Muffins

Serves 4-6

Prep: 10 minutes
Bake: 15 minutes
Let Stand: 5 minutes

Ingredients:

- Three 6oz. cans chunk white albacore (dolphin free) tuna OR if looking to make *vegetarian you can use one 16 oz. can of chickpeas/garbanzo beans, drained and mashed with a fork or masher
- 4-6 oz. shredded Swiss cheese or vegan cheese
- 12 slices whole wheat or multigrain bread, crusts cut off
- 2-3 T olive oil OR organic butter
- 2-3 T mayonnaise or vegan mayo
- 1 t curry powder (a little more or less depending on taste)
- 2 T dried cranberries or raisins
- Non-stick olive oil cooking spray
- Salt & pepper to taste

Directions:

- Preheat oven to 375 degrees. Coat muffin tray (for 12 muffins) with cooking spray.
- Drizzle or lightly brush one side of bread with olive oil or a little butter and press oil side up into muffin cups.
- In a bowl combine tuna or mashed chickpeas, 1 T olive oil, mayo, cheese, curry powder, cranberries or raisins, and salt & pepper to taste. Mix well. (Add more mayo/curry etc. to taste)
- Divide mixture into each bread-lined muffin cup.
- Top with shredded cheese.
- Bake for 15 minutes or until filling is bubbly hot and top browning.

Idea: Serve with a green salad and chopped apple on the side.

Sweet and Sexy Kale Salad

Serves: 2

Ingredients:

- 4-6 cups washed and dried finely chopped Kale
- 1 cup cherry tomatoes, (go for mix of red and yellow for extra flavor) sliced in half
- ½ cup feta cheese
- ¼ cup dried cranberries
- 1 green apple cut into small strips
- ¼ cup walnuts, broken into pieces
- Sea salt and pepper to taste

Dressing:

Apple Cider Vinaigrette:

- 2 T olive oil
- 1 T apple cider vinegar
- 1 T dijon mustard
- Whisk all together in a bowl until creamy.

Directions:

- Mix all together in a bowl and toss with dressing.

Veggie Burger with Apple Cider Vinaigrette

Serves: One

This warm veggie sandwich is great for a quick lunch or a snack.

Keep a stash of veggie burgers in the freezer so you can whip one up anytime.

Ingredients:

- 2 slices sprouted grain or whole grain bread
- 1-2 Tbs olive
- One frozen veggie patty/burger (Check labels to find a brand that's right for you like Amy's Kitchen or Dr. Praeger's)
- Sliced avocado
- Sliced mushrooms
- Spinach leaves or salad greens
- Sliced cheese or vegan cheese (optional)

Dressing:

- 1 T cider vinegar
- 1 T Dijon mustard
- 2 T olive oil
- Whisk all together in a small bowl

Directions:

- Toast bread.
- Heat oil in skillet and cook patty.
- Moisten toast with a little olive oil then drizzle on dressing.
- Add patty and start building your sandwich with veggies.

- Drizzle on the rest of dressing.
- If adding cheese, leave off top half of bread and melt cheese under broiler or in toaster oven.
- Add a pinch of salt and pepper and add remaining bread.
- Serve with some fresh cut seasonal veggies on the side.

Chicken Breasts With Tomato, Basil & Arugula/Spinach

This easy, healthy recipe for boneless chicken breasts with fresh tomatoes, basil and arugula and/or spinach will become one of your favorite dishes for friends and family!

Serves 4

Prep time: 15 minutes
Cook time: Approx. 20 minutes

Ingredients:

- 4 Organic, skinless, boneless chicken breasts (about 1.5 to 2 lbs)
- ¼-½ cup thinly sliced packed fresh basil leaves
- 1 lb ripe tomatoes (plum, beefsteak, whatever looks fresh and preferably local) diced into ½-inch cubes.
- 4-6 cups baby arugula or spinach (or a combination of both- washed and air or spun dry)
- 5-6 T. extra-virgin olive oil
- 2.5 T. balsamic vinegar
- 1-2 cloves garlic, finely chopped
- Sea salt and freshly ground black pepper to taste

Directions:

- Wash and pat dry chicken breasts and season with salt and pepper.
- Heat 2 T of the oil in large skillet over medium-high heat until just shimmering.

- Cook chicken on one side for 8-10 minutes (depending on how thick breasts are) until golden-brown then flip and continue to cook on other side another 8-10 minutes, scraping together any brown bits. (Add a little extra olive oil if needed and cook a few minutes longer if needed at a medium heat—always check to make sure chicken is cooked thoroughly!)

As the chicken is cooking:

- In a medium size bowl, combine tomatoes, basil, garlic, vinegar, 3 Tbs oil and about ¼ t salt and pepper (to taste)
- Let the chicken cool a few minutes then slice into 2-inch strips (or you can serve the breasts whole, whatever you fancy!)
- On a large platter make a bed with the arugula or spinach mixture
- Arrange the chicken on top and spoon on the tomato mixture and drizzle the juice over all.

'Creamy' Spinach Soup

You won't believe how creamy this vegan soup is. It is so healthy, delicious and 'creamy' without the cream! Full of fresh spinach, zucchini, and cauliflower, it's sure to become one of your favorites and it's so easy to make.

Serves: 8

Prep: 15 mins
Cook Time: 45 mins total

Ingredients:

- 1-2 T olive oil
- 1 large onion, diced
- 3 cloves garlic, sliced thin
- 3 zucchini, quartered and cut into ½-inch pieces
- 1 large potato, diced
- 1 head cauliflower, washed and chopped or broken into pieces
- 3-4 cups tightly packed spinach (washed, dried, stems removed)
- 8 cups low-sodium organic vegetable broth
- Sea salt and pepper to taste

Directions:

- Add olive oil to preheated soup pot.
- Add onion and cook over medium heat for 5-10 minutes until translucent (Don't let it brown.)

- Add sliced garlic and continue to cook for another 5 minutes.
- Add zucchini and continue cooking another 5 minutes or so, stirring to mix.
- Add vegetable broth, potatoes and cauliflower and bring to boil and simmer for about 30 minutes. (Until potato and
- cauliflower pieces are completely cooked and soft to touch.)
- Add spinach leaves, stirring in and cook another 3-5 minutes.

To Complete:

- Transfer broth mixture to a blender, immersion blender or food processor. Puree all of the ingredients together (I like to use my immersion blender so I keep all the action right in the soup pot.)
- Return mixture to pot if using blender/food processor, and adjust seasoning, adding salt and pepper as desired.

(This soup heats up well so you can enjoy it for a few days!)

Asian Stir-Fry with Zucchini Noodles

Serves: 4

Ingredients: *(note: you can omit the chicken and add in another cup of veggies for vegetarian/vegan option)*

Ingredients:

- 1.5 lbs organic chicken breasts cut into bite-size pieces
- 2-4 T olive oil
- 3 cloves chopped garlic
- 1 red onion, chopped
- 3-4 cups chopped broccoli, carrots, cauliflower, red pepper, and/or mushrooms

  (You can get creative here and add veggies that you like or have on hand. Think about adding green beans, snow peas, chopped bok choy, etc.)
- 3 T grated fresh ginger
- one small can well-drained water chestnuts (optional)
- ¼-½ cup Tamari organic low-sodium soy sauce (you can use another brand, but this one is so tasty)
- 1-2 T organic brown sugar (optional, but really adds a nice 'sweet' and sour taste and per serving still keeps it very low in sugar)
- Juice of ½ lemon (optional)
- 3 medium to large zucchini (for 'noodles')
- 1 finely sliced green onion top for garnish

Note: *for gluten free option, use Bragg's liquid aminos or use a gluten free soy sauce*

Directions:

- In medium bowl add chicken and 2 T grated ginger and stir to coat with 2-4 T of the soy sauce. Set aside.
- In large skillet, heat about 2 T of the olive oil until just shimmering.
- Add garlic and red onion and cook 3-5 minutes, making sure it doesn't burn.
- Add mixed veggies and cook over medium heat another 5 minutes, stirring occasionally and adding a little more oil if needed and a few splashes of soy sauce. (Make sure to not 'burn' or brown the veggies, you want them to stay a little crisp.)
- Push the veggies around to the outer edges of the pan and add chicken to the middle.
- Let chicken sit and cook in the middle for 3-5 minutes.
- Begin to move and mix the chicken and veggies together, adding in a few more splashes of soy sauce. Add in a little more oil if needed.
- Continue cooking another 5-7 minutes (or until chicken is cooked through) stirring gently.
- Add in the remaining ginger and sprinkle in the sugar (if adding) and stir it all up.
- Squeeze the lemon over all ingredients if you like.
- Add sea salt and pepper to taste. (TIP: Be aware that the soy sauce can be salty, so taste before adding the salt.)

For Zucchini Noodles:

Using a mandoline slicer with a julienne blade. Slice zucchini lengthwise into 'noodles.' Or use a knife to cut it lengthwise into thin noodle like strips or you can use a vegetable peeler. Steam or sauté until tender, about 3-5 minutes. These noodles are great as a substitute for pasta and other recipes.

To Serve:

Serve stir-fry over bed of zucchini noodles and sprinkle with green onions.

Black Bean and Corn Chili

Serves: 6

Ingredients:

(Please note: there is a vegetarian option, a red meat option or white meat option)

- 1 and ¼ lbs ground organic ground sirloin, turkey or chicken OR if going total vegetarian one can of red kidney beans, drained and rinsed
- 1 large onion, chopped (reserve two T for garnish, if desired)
- 3-4 cloves garlic, minced
- 2 T olive oil
- 1-15 oz can organic black beans, drained and rinsed
- 1-15 oz. can organic whole kernel corn, drained
- 1-28 oz. can chopped tomatoes
- 1-15 oz. can tomato sauce
- ½ t ground cumin
- 3 T chili powder
- 2-3 T dried oregano
- ¼ t salt
- 1-2 T dark brown sugar (depending on sweet you like it)
- Dash cayenne (to taste)
- 1-2 cups prepared brown rice or quinoa according to package directions to serve chili over. *Tip: Try using vegetable broth instead of water for more flavor.*

For garnish:

- Reserved chopped onion
- ¼ cup chopped fresh cilantro (optional)
- Sour cream
- Shredded cheese/vegan cheese

Directions:

- Heat oil in large, heavy bottom soup-style pan.
- Cook onion and garlic about 5 minutes, making sure not to brown, until onion is clear
- Add 2 T oregano (crush with palms to release flavor) Stir with onion and garlic and cook another minute.
- Add *meat and break apart into pan, stirring all together *(IF adding meat, if not, continue directions and add can of red beans when adding the black beans.)
- Cook approx. 8 minutes, stirring and blending.
- Cook until meat is done then drain off any excess fat that has accumulated.
- Add tomatoes and tomato sauce, stirring all together.
- Add all remaining dry seasonings keeping in mind you can always adjust seasonings as you go. (Go light on the cayenne until you've given it the taste test)
- Simmer at low heat another 3-5 minutes.
- Add in beans and corn, continue to simmer several more minutes, blending all together gently.
- Taste and add one T dark brown sugar at a time if you'd like it a little sweeter. Do this by stirring it into chili with a wooden spoon for several minutes for it to dissolve.
- Continue to simmer and adjust seasonings, adding in more salt, sugar, oregano, cayenne, etc. if needed.

Serve over brown rice or quinoa, garnish with cilantro, onion, sour cream and/or cheese and serve with a nice green side salad full of fresh veggies.

Baked Salmon Teriyaki With Sautéed Baby Bok Choy with Garlic & Ginger

Serves: 4

Note: Salmon needs several hours to marinate.
Cook quinoa or brown rice as a nice companion for a complete meal.

Ingredients for Salmon:

- 4 (6 ounce) salmon steaks
- ¼ cup sesame oil (If you don't have on hand, use olive oil)
- ¼ cup lemon juice
- ¼ cup organic low-sodium soy sauce like Tamari (or gluten free soy sauce)
- 2 T's brown sugar, or more to taste OR 2-3 t honey.
- 1 T sesame seeds
- 1 t fresh dijon mustard or ground mustard
- 1 t ground ginger
- 1-2 cloves minced garlic or one t garlic powder
- 4 lemon slices for garnish (optional)

Directions:

- Mix oil, lemon juice, soy sauce, brown sugar/honey, sesame seeds, mustard, ginger, and garlic powder in a small saucepan over low heat.
- Bring to a simmer, stirring until sugar has dissolved.
- Set aside ½ cup of marinade for basting.
- Let cool for a few minutes then pour remaining marinade into a re-sealable plastic bag and place salmon into the marinade.

- Squeeze excess air out of the bag, seal, and marinate the salmon steaks for at least 2 hours. Drain and discard used marinade.
- Place oven rack about 4-inches from the heat source and preheat the oven's broiler.
- Put salmon steaks into a broiler pan and broil for 5 minutes.
- Brush with reserved marinade, turn, and broil until fish is opaque and flakes easily, about 5 more minutes.
- Baste again with marinade.

Sautéed Baby Bok Choy with Garlic and Ginger

Serves: 4

Ingredients:

- 4-5 bunches of baby bok choy OR 2 large bunches, chopped and rinsed well *(they can be gritty so make sure to pull apart leaves and rinse well.)*
- 1 T olive oil
- 4 garlic cloves, smashed
- 2 slices of fresh ginger, peeled and smashed (optional)
- sea salt and pepper to taste
- 1 T (splash) of organic low-sodium soy sauce (or liquid aminos or gluten free soy sauce)

Directions:

- Heat the oil in heavy bottom skillet or wok pan.
- Add garlic and cook for 4-5 minutes.
- Add bok choy and ginger and cook until tender, stirring and coating all.
- Add a splash or two of the soy sauce.
- Season with sea salt and pepper to taste.

Prepare 1 cup brown rice or quinoa according to package directions. **Plate salmon, Bok Choy and rice or quinoa for a delicious meal!**

CHAPTER 8:

Putting it Into Practice to Make it A Reality

For those of you still doubting if investing in yourself is better than investing in gimmicks and pills; this chapter is a must read for you. Brian's transformation highlights just how important changing your mindset is when it comes to food and drinking.

I wanted to end the book with his story because I think it is truly inspirational and illustrates how changing your mindset, habits and behaviors will impact so much more than the number in the scale. You will feel the impact forever in your everyday life.

Brian

Brian started to work with me after his wife purchased a 2-hour V.I.P Day special that I was running. Brian filled out my questionnaire and sent me food records followed by a 2-hour Skype session.

I gathered all of my information about Brian, his goals, his past and current diet history, exercise, medical and present lifestyle information and created a personalized nutrition plan for him. At the time, Brian wasn't interested in doing a longer-term program. He thought all he needed was a plan.

About three months later I received an email from Brian asking about my 6-month program. He wanted to lose 30 lbs, and he realized that he couldn't do it without the guidance, accountability and support I could provide. In our first few meetings, we talked about Brian's work and home life. We found there were habits and behaviors he had established that were not only contributing to his weight but that over time, would cause issues with his health. Brian was a lawyer and had three young children. Needless to say, he had a very busy and at times, a stressful life. Having young kids there were always snacks on hand which sometimes went along with some wine or some bourbon he used to unwind after a long day when the kids went to sleep. Though not thrilled at the thought of changing this night-time ritual, he was happy to give it a go. What he really had a hard time with was the idea of not drinking at client dinners or business events when traveling. He assumed that he 'just wouldn't be able to.'

Brian was an excellent example of someone who took our coaching conversations and really thought about the work in-between our meetings. He asked himself the right questions when he used his self-talk, and he thought about what he was getting, NOT what he was giving up. As he began to sleep better, have more energy and have a sense of overall wellness, his mindset and lifestyle changes became easier and easier. AND...I am happy to share that by the time we were done, Brian had no problem not drinking at home and limiting his drinks while out from zero to three at most. Yup! Brian was able to go out for business dinners and events and, if he had it in his mind, not have a drink at all. I think he was even surprised at his ability to do so.

Here is what Brian had to say about his journey to transformation:

I am 5'7" and 51 years old. When I first met with Lisa Goldberg in [December 2015], I weighed about 175 pounds. As I write this in June 2016, I weigh about 145 pounds. The difference is insignificant in a way (not exactly Biggest Loser numbers, after all), but the effect on how I feel, what I can do, how well my body handles exercise and activities with my kids, is almost indescribable.

This reward is sweet; it took time and commitment, and I earned it. So, it is empowering in that way that success is. It's a peculiar sort of accomplishment though. It did not require great intelligence or athleticism, or talent, or education, or experience; in that respect, it is a reward attainable by almost anyone. But when I started, I had no idea how to go about it. I knew I weighed more than I should, although I did not really understand why. I did not always weigh too much, but habits that I managed easily in my 20s and even my 30s were now taking a toll. And, it would only get worse as I aged; my ability to burn energy through exercise would continue to diminish over time. So, I knew the solution to long-term health lay in what I ate and drank. But I had no idea how to tackle it.

The first step for me was deciding I really wanted to make this change. This seems obvious, and even easy in November when you decide you want to do it later, after the holidays... But here is what I was facing:

1. *I love eating and drinking. So any change to what I ate and drank was going to have an immediate negative impact, requiring me to change something I love doing, right now.*

2. *The benefits of these changes would not be felt immediately. So, in the near term, I was facing deprivation without reward.*

3. *I had no idea how to go about eating better. Just by way of simple example, if I were busy at work and carved out 30 minutes to get lunch, I would have no idea where to get anything other than a sandwich. Vegetables and other items did not even register in my brain stem as food.*

What I needed was a coach- someone who could give me some direction and structure, to whom I would be accountable.

Before I even met with Lisa, she asked me to complete a questionnaire that provided her with a snapshot of where I was with food: what foods I ate, what I drank, how often, what I didn't like and similar matters. I then met with her via Skype for about an hour so she could develop a complete profile, following which she sent me some specific recommendations for food options, appropriate portion sizes, and similar matters. We talked at some length about one of my major logistical concerns. Where would I find the right food (particularly since most of my meals are purchased near my office from sandwich shops, or are business meals taken at restaurants)? And, Lisa surprised me with some specific ideas in my neighborhood about which she had first- hand knowledge. As follow up to the Skype session, Lisa sent me a written summary along with a comprehensive list of food (and even some restaurant) options, which were likely to be more palatable to me based on my profile. I now had information I could use to start making changes.

I could have left it there, and for a short while I tried to put this information to work on my own; but not surprisingly, I did almost nothing with it. I realized the information by itself was not enough; I needed someone to give me a push, to account to on a regular basis, to be my 'food conscience' until I could develop one on my own. I decided to commit to several months of personal coaching with Lisa.

At our first session, Lisa handed me a book called 'Savor - Mindful Eating, Mindful Life.' I won't review the book, and in fact, I stopped reading after the first chapter (when it became somewhat preachy; after all, my personal objective was not to save the planet by becoming a vegan). But the underlying philosophy conveyed the first several pages was straightforward and compelling: be mindful of what you eat and drink. I realized, as I read and absorbed this, that very much of my eating and drinking was habitual and without any regard for the benefits or costs regarding how it would make me feel. Sitting down in the evening to watch a ballgame with random snacks and cocktails was pretty standard. I very much enjoyed these rituals, and many others involving food and drink, but my consumption had no relation to how hungry I was or what it was doing for me.

Similarly, I had no idea how much food I needed to eat at mealtimes to fill me up. So the default answer was to eat for as long as the food lasted (I was a platinum member of the clean plate club at restaurants, with the exception of most vegetables), or as long as people were still eating.

Lisa had already provided me with data on this, but it was much more useful when I started learning how to think about food.

Mindful eating. I really cannot stress enough how powerful this quasi-mnemonic can be. In simple terms, it has allowed me to learn how much food I need to eat, and how to choose the right foods and quantities. I now feel OK leaving part of a meal unfinished. I don't feel compelled to eat what my kids left on their plates or to eat the last half of a cheeseburger so it won't go to waste. I can easily choose to watch the ballgame and not mindlessly grind through a bag of chips.

More generally, I can choose to make meals out of good food. Over time, vegetables have become food to my primitive brain, and I like them. This doesn't mean I like all of them all the time (I'm still not a vegan). And it doesn't mean I still don't like other things including steak, cheese and, yes, chips and beer. In fact, Lisa stressed from the very beginning that I was NOT on a 'diet' that would prohibit me from eating anything I wanted; rather,

I was developing a more active relationship with food that would allow me to choose when and how much I would have of anything I wanted. So, a holiday barbecue still can include a hamburger and apple pie; but I am much more likely now to include a salad, and skip the extra hot dog. The key is thinking about it, making an active choice, among real options, armed with knowledge about what and how much I really need, and how much of what I don't need I can allow myself to have anyway.

Lisa also has been a great coach. Before I could develop my own inner monolog about food, I needed an external voice. During our time together I recorded my eating and reported daily to Lisa. She doesn't tell me what to eat, but occasionally asks the sort of question I should be asking myself (such as, are you aware you had ten glasses of wine in 3 days?). Now, these are questions I ask myself, and usually, I do it ahead of time before I head out for the evening so that I can plan ahead. But at the beginning, I was not equipped to engage in this sort of thought process, and having someone like Lisa to train with in the beginning was crucial.

One other specific topic merits discussion in my case: alcohol. When I decided to try to change my eating, I knew I could not ignore my consumption of alcohol. I love drinking. I love the ritual around sharing a good bottle of wine, a glass of great bourbon, a beer at a ballgame ... I knew unlimited drinking was counterproductive to my overall goal, but I also was skeptical about my ability to reduce the amount I was drinking. (I did not really know how much that was, but in retrospect, I was probably averaging 3 or 4 drinks a day). But, the 'mindfulness' mnemonic really is a powerful tool. Over time, I have reduced my alcohol consumption to about one drink per day. This has meant several days a week without drinking (so no more drinking alone at home...), and other days when I will have 1 or 2 drinks (occasionally, but rarely, 3). I don't really miss the extra drinks; it has turned out most of those were not necessary for me to enjoy the ritual and social aspects of drinking, but rather were just excess volume I didn't need and didn't really enjoy that much after all. (As an aside, I was relieved to confirm that I did not have a physical addiction to alcohol; I won't pretend the act of being mindful could have addressed that sort of problem; my guess is that it wouldn't.)

So several months after getting started, I feel better than I have in years, I get better sleep, have more energy, enjoy better workouts, and (according to several biased family members) look 20 years younger than I did at the start. More important, I believe these changes reflect a new, permanent relationship with food that I can sustain, rather than some crash period of deprivation that would inevitably reverse itself. The only problem is that none of my clothes fit anymore. In the overall scheme of things, I consider that a high- class problem.

Brian lost five more pounds by the time we were done and met his 30lb weight loss goal. He not only changed his weight- he changed his mindset which helped him change his lifestyle.

Ironically, as I am finishing this book I sat with a client who was finishing her program. She lost 20 lbs, and she looked great! During our conversation I was telling her to be aware of Cocky Dieters Syndrome, (as discussed in Chapter 4) to stay mindful and to remember all of the tools and strategies she has under her belt. Most important is to remember the hard work she put into changing her habits and behaviors. This MUST continue to maintain the weight loss. She agreed saying "it's really about a way of living." I reminded her "it's really about a way of thinking so you can stay living a healthy lifestyle."

A Few Final Words

I know there is a lot of information in this book, and I hope much of it resonated with you. I hope you are feeling excited about starting your journey to sustainable weight loss, but I do recognize you may be feeling a bit nervous or overwhelmed at getting started.

Take a deep breathe and start to slowly manage your mindset. Believe you can do this. Trust yourself. And most of all remember your WHY. Put sticky notes all over your home and or office to remind you of your new self-talk and your new messaging. Treat yourself to a new datebook where you can schedule YOU in. Book dates with yourself and plan everything else around that. Practicing self-care is not selfish but self-preservation. If you are your best self, you will show up better for everyone else in your life.

Take it slow. It's your journey and slow and steady wins the race.

If you want to share your wins with me I would love to hear from you. Please drop me a line at lisa@lisagoldbergnutrition.com.

As a special gift to you for purchasing <u>Food Fight</u> I am including a link to one of my webinars 4 Mindset Strategies for Sustainable Weight Loss. http://events.instantteleseminar.com/?eventid=87241548

To good Health & Happy Days!

XO,

Lisa

Made in the USA
Middletown, DE
18 May 2017